Nature to the Rescue!

How to Build
Your Own
Herbal First Aid Kit

Nature to the Rescue!
How to Build Your Own
Herbal First Aid Kit

Printed in the United States of America
ISBN: 978-1481166058

Cover Design by: Diane Kidman

Published by: carp(e) libris press, LLC

Visit the Author Website at:
www.DianeKidman.com

Table of Contents

Introduction

Remember last summer when your husband was teaching the kids to skateboard on the driveway? Everything was going fine until he attempted that Ollie, something he never could do right, even back when he had good knees and 20/20 vision. The kids still claim he took a dive with such finesse and air lift that even Shaun White would have been impressed. All you remember is the gash on your husband's forehead, an impressive looking laceration that made your stomach flop when you saw it. But you knew what to do. You ran for the first aid kit you always keep stocked and ready under the bathroom sink.

Oh, wait. You didn't have a first aid kit. In fact, if I move your strategically placed oriental throw rug, I can still see the remnants of your husband's blood donation to the living room floor.

Thankfully, your husband came out of it with nothing more than a thin scar and bragging rights for life. But ever since then, you've been telling yourself to get that first aid kit together and be ready because Junior takes after his father in the grace department.

1

What You'll be Learning

You're about to embark on an herbal journey, one that will give you the opportunity to prepare and use your own natural medicines. The first part of this book is organized by emergency. You'll learn about various herbal remedies and preparations for each situation. From these suggestions, you can decide which remedies you'll want to include in your own kit. If an emergency does arise, just flip to the *Find it Fast* section of each chapter where you'll find quick instructions on how to use your homemade remedies, along with when it's best to call for emergency help.

Toward the end of the book, you'll find the step-by-step instructions on how to make the salves, tinctures, and medicinal oils needed to complete your herbal first aid kit. You'll also learn what other supplies should be added to make the kit complete.

If there's one thing I've discovered when talking to readers, it's that there are a great many people out there who have a desire to learn herbalism and to make their family's medicinal choices more natural, but they're held back from doing things on their own because the information seems daunting and complicated. Don't worry. We'll break things down nice and simple. You can get more complicated later on if you like, but remember that medicinal herbs have been relied on since the beginning of humankind, and those early cave dwellers didn't do very well with rocket science.

Information to Keep with Your Kit

A printed copy of the book "First Aid/CPR/AED Participant's Manual" by the American Red Cross is an excellent addition to your kit. It can be purchased through the American Red Cross website (www.redcross.org), or you can download it in PDF format for free at http://editiondigital.net/publication/?i=64159. If you opt for the free PDF, be sure to print out a clear copy and store it with the kit. You can also store it on your personal electronic devices so it's always handy. While it's a hefty 200 pages, it's a worthwhile read on everything from CPR and AED (automated external defibrillator) to broken bones and heart attacks.

The Red Cross also has an app called "First Aid App" that

you can keep on your phone or tablet. It contains step-by-step instructions and enables you to connect directly to your local emergency service.

If you've purchased "Nature to the Rescue!" as an ebook, it is also available in paperback and can be kept with your kit for easier reference.

Bites & Stings

I consider myself an expert of sorts in the bite and sting department. That's because I've been bitten and stung more than my share of times. Perhaps I should be used to it by now, but I still don't take it very gracefully. One time I was able to put these remedies to the test, it was beneath an additional layer of duress. My son, who was about four at the time, was trotting behind me on the way to the mailbox. Right as we got there, he fell down and scraped up his forearms on the sidewalk. I scooped him up and grabbed the mailbox door, which had grown a small hornet's nest overnight. I also grabbed three hornets who weren't happy I squished their house. Within a few seconds, my son and I were both wailing. Before I even got back to the house, my hand was throbbing and swollen, my son's forearms seeping blood around bits of embedded gravel.

At times like this, it's hard to remember all the things you'd usually know. We all have remedies we recommend to friends like we're old pros, but when the injury occurs (especially to one of our children) all those sage words seem to fly away. Yet another reason to keep your first aid kit ready before you need it. Sometimes a trip to the mailbox results in more than a fresh stack of junk mail.

The following remedies are the ones I remember to use once I get myself together a bit. One of them you already have in your kitchen. The others are simple items that will become important staples to your herbal first aid kit.

Bite & Sting Remedies

The most basic and reliable insect sting remedy I know isn't even an herb. But you probably already have some, so let's get it added to your first aid kit. **Baking soda** is excellent for drawing out the venom of an insect sting or any nasty bug bite. Keep a small tin or container of baking soda in your kit. A teaspoon of baking soda is mixed with water to form a paste. Make sure it's not too sloppy, but you do want some moisture there. If it's too dry and crumbly, it won't work. Place a thick layer of the paste on the wound and allow it to thoroughly dry. The sooner you can make use of this remedy, the better. I've found that if I can use it within the first minutes after the sting has occurred, the pain will subside and the skin will look as though it was never attacked in the first place.

I've even used this remedy on one of my dachshunds who got stung by a wasp (at least I *think* that's what she said). I wasn't sure where the sting was, so I just coated her whole leg in paste. I got lots of nose licks for that one.

A good partner to the baking soda is **echinacea** (*Echinacea angustifolia* or *purpurea*). It's helpful in cases of insect stings and spider bites when taken internally, as it cools the body down and relieves swollen membranes. This is an especially good choice for children.

The thought of a spider bite or a scorpion sting give us all a case of the willies, but learning how to deal with them can reduce our fears. In actuality, very few spiders can bite a human because those jaws are too tiny to grab our skin. But there are a few who can, and do, bite people. Spiders such as the black widow and the brown recluse are venomous, and while they don't have the poison to kill the average person, they are particularly dangerous to the very young, the elderly, and the infirm.

Native Americans once viewed echinacea first and foremost as a remedy for spider, scorpion, and even snake bites.

Echinacea (*Echinacea angustifolia* and *purpurea*) should be given in tincture form to help combat the side effects of these bites.

Plantain (*Plantago major* or *minor*) excels at drawing out poisons and foreign objects, and it's readily available in most backyards, fields, and forests throughout the U.S., Mexico, Europe, Australia, and much of Canada and South America. (Check www.eol.org for a series of photos and distribution maps, and be sure of proper identification before picking your own. Also, never use chemically treated, fertilized, or sprayed plants.) It can even be dug up out of the snow, which makes it especially handy year round. While you can store plantain salve in your first aid kit (you'll learn how to make your own later), the fresh leaves are superior. You can smash the fresh leaves in a mortar and pestle before applying to the wound and covering with gauze.

Find it Fast

Bee and Insect Stings, Spider Bites: Mix one teaspoon of baking soda with enough water to make a thick but wet paste. Apply to the sting and allow to dry thoroughly; rinse and repeat if needed.

NOTE: This remedy does NOT replace proper emergency care for those who are allergic to bee stings.

Mosquito Bites: Apply plantain salve liberally to the affected area. If fresh leaves are available, smash well with a mortar and pestle, or crush a leaf and rub it on the bite until the skin turns green from the leaf juice. Repeat either form as needed.

Spider Bites, Scorpion Stings, and Other Venomous Bites: Wash affected area thoroughly with soap and water. Apply a fresh plantain leaf poultice if you have the plantain leaves available to you. Cover the poultice with gauze and change regularly until the area has calmed down. Follow either treatment with 30 to 100 drops of echinacea tincture, to be given as soon as possible. Continue dose every one to two hours for several hours thereafter. At this point, keep the sting or bite uncovered for proper drainage. Be sure to seek immediate medical attention if the bite or sting came from a dangerously venomous creature and the bitten individual is either young, elderly, or infirm.

When to Call 9-1-1

- Shoulder, chest, back, or abdomen muscles become rigid.
- Restlessness, headache, weakness, dizziness, anxiety, and/or excessive sweating is present.
- Eyelids swell up or appear droopy.
- When severe pain or cramping is present, especially in abdomen or back.
- Chills, fever, nausea, and/or vomiting.
- Trouble breathing, swallowing.
- Chest pain and/or elevated heart rate.

Breathing

Whether it's caused by asthma, pneumonia, bronchitis, or exposure to pollutants, breathing problems need attention fast. Your lungs definitely deserve a solid herbal remedy or two within your kit. If someone is having trouble breathing, it's never something to mess around with. Have these tea blends ready to go ahead of time, especially if you have someone in your household with asthma or other breathing issues, or if bronchitis or pneumonia visit your family often. Herbal remedies like the ones to follow can do a lot to open the lungs, but asthmatics should use their emergency inhalers or other doctor prescribed emergency medications first, before attempting herbal medications. The following tea blends are normally safe to use in conjunction with prescription asthma inhalers, but be sure to check with your doctor or pharmacist ahead of time so you know if these blends are safe for you.

Breathing Remedies

If someone in your home is having trouble breathing but you don't feel it's an emergency, these teas should help reverse the problem. If you do have an emergency on your hands, of course call 9-1-1 first. Then, while waiting for that help, you can prepare a strong tea of the following dried herbs: 1 part **mullein** leaf (*Verbascum thapsus*), 1 part **white pine bark** (*Pinus spp.*), 1 part **licorice** root (*Glycyrrhiza glabra*). Or try my special tea blend outlined in the Find it Fast section. My own blend may not have the best of flavors, I'll admit; but it will clear the lungs of mucus while reducing the inflammation.

Blend these herbs ahead of time and store them in a small marked and dated jar within your kit. These teas are appropriate for asthma, bronchitis, pneumonia, and many other lung issues. When a breathing problem strikes, shake the jar to blend the herbs and prepare the tea. Chewing a raw piece of ginger can also open the lungs and is a quick remedy while waiting for the tea to steep.

Find it Fast

Mullein Leaf Blend: Combine one part dried mullein leaf, one part dried white pine bark, and one part dried licorice root (cut for tea). Steep two teaspoons of the blend per one cup of hot water for 15 to 20 minutes. Strain and drink as needed.

Diane's Lung Relief Blend: Combine one part of each of the following dried herbs: Mullein leaf, white pine bark, licorice root, wild cherry bark, marshmallow root, horehound root, elecampane root, and spearmint leaves. Steep two teaspoons of the blend per one cup of hot water for 20 to 25 minutes. Strain and drink as needed.

When to Call 9-1-1
- Breathing is labored and causes pain in the chest, tingling sensations in the hands, the feet, or the lips.
- Wheezing, high-pitched sounds, or gurgling noises coming from the chest.
- Gasping for breath.
- Shallow breathing, rapid breathing, or the breathing has stopped entirely.

In general, breathing that is too fast, too slow, causes pain, or makes noise requires emergency help. Until help arrives, keep the person seated upright, as this usually allows for freer breathing than does lying down. Make sure any restrictive clothing is released. Breathing difficulties feel scary and usually cause fear and anxiety in those experiencing it. Reassuring words and a calm, relaxed attitude on your part will be helpful.

Bruises

I can never figure out where my bruises come from, other than a vague memory of pain the day before. Either I bruise easily or I'm so distracted that having a bowling ball dropped on my thigh isn't enough to garner my attention. Whether you remember receiving that nasty bruise or not, you can treat it with herbs. Yes, the ever popular ice pack is always a good option. But add an herb or two, and you might still be able to wear nylons to the Christmas party.

Bruise Remedies

Good for both skin abrasions and bruises, the herb **hyssop** (*Hyssopus officinalis*) makes a fine tea to be used topically. It's also antiviral and antispasmodic, so if any cuts or muscle pain accompanied your bump, you'll find relief. **Calendula** (*Calendula officinalis*) can also be used and has the added benefit of reducing the risk of scarring if an open cut is present. Its anti-inflammatory , antibacterial, and antiviral properties are among its star qualities, not to mention its pain relieving abilities when being used externally.

Our friend **peppermint** (*Mentha piperita*) makes yet another appearance. This circulatory stimulant also relieves muscle spasms and muscle tension when applied topically. Alternatively, a banged up and stressed out individual can drink the tea to ease the tension that often comes with any bruise inducing activities. Like falling out of bed. That's never good.

While you can't store **ice packs** in your first aid kit, you should always have something ready and waiting in the freezer. Alternatively, disposable **instant compress packs** are available for first aid kits and work for hours when squeezed and shaken. Either version is imperative. After my son took a spill down a few steps and went head first onto a concrete basement floor, I ran him up the stairs as fast as I could and plopped an ice pack on his head within seconds. What started out as a scary trip to Urgent Care resulted in nothing more than a minor bruise to the noggin. I accredit the ice pack with his quick recovery. We kept the pack on the bruise from the house to the Urgent Care facility, through the one-hour wait (in an empty waiting room, I might add). The doctor said my son would have a big lump and a nasty bruise by the looks of things, but by the next day, the spot was barely noticeable. The wonders of a basic remedy!

Find it Fast

Hyssop, Calendula, or Peppermint: Steep one teaspoon of dried herb in a cup of hot water for 15 to 20 minutes. When cool enough for comfort, apply topically as needed.

Ice Packs or Instant Compress Packs: Immediately applying ice packs, instant cold compresses, even a bag of frozen peas to a bruised or banged sight can greatly reduce swelling, pain, and recovery time, not to mention reducing the size and intensity of the resulting bruise.

When to Call 9-1-1

- Severe pain or an inability to move a body part without pain.
- The force that caused injury seemed strong enough to have caused serious damage.
- Vomiting blood or the coughing up of blood.
- Confusion, drowsiness, dizziness, shock, or unconsciousness.
- A pale or blue extremity.
- A distended and/or tender abdomen.

Note: Apply ice packs to injured area while awaiting emergency help.

Burns

There's that old idiom "Experience is the best teacher." Makes you wonder why most of us still get burned in the kitchen. Alas, cooking is one of the most common ways to receive a burn, hence a good array of burn remedies will become an essential part of your herbal first aid kit. But not all the remedies will be boxed up.

My mother, for instance, always had an aloe plant in the kitchen, so to me it's just part of a cook's wares. I currently have an aloe plant so large that it has to sit on the floor, but I'm glad to have so much of it. I doubt there's a leaf on it that hasn't already been pinched off, whether it was to care for someone's sunburn or to soothe my own scorched hand after picking up an iron skillet without a potholder.

Burn Remedies

Of course, an aloe plant doesn't fit into the case of a first aid kit very neatly, but it is my number one remedy for all kinds of burns. These inexpensive houseplants are easy to maintain and require little water (overwatering results in weaker gel), so I recommend getting one for your home. If you want to add a store bought bottle of aloe gel to your first aid kit, make sure it's as natural as possible. The popular bright neon green gels sold in most stores are not natural; just check out those ingredients. Aloe vera is probably somewhere on the list, but it's buried under preservatives, colorants, and alcohols. Even the most natural brands contain additives, so be sure that if you choose to purchase bottled gel it contains only a small list of ingredients. The best brands contain only natural additives. And they don't glow in the dark.

Aloe (*Aloe vera*) works for sunburns, 1st, 2nd, and 3rd degree burns, and has even been used with success on radiation burns. If you're using a plant, choose the flatter and older looking leaves. Those contain strongly hypertonic gel that will work more effectively at drawing excess fluid from your burn and into the leaves.

To use the leaves, cut or peel them open lengthwise and place them directly on the wound. For smaller burns such as the kind one might get while cooking, pinch the end of an aloe leaf off the plant and squeeze the gel onto the burn. You can store the leaf in an airtight container in the refrigerator for later reapplication.

Another burn remedy is calendula oil. **Calendula** (*Calendula officinalis*) assists skin in the granulation process. Granulation is what happens when the skin heals itself by filling in an injury with fresh new tissue called "granulation tissue." The tissue is pink and often uneven and damp, and it can benefit from calendula as a follow-up treatment for all burns. Calendula is very useful for many kinds of injuries, so be sure to include some in your kit. Instructions for preparation can be found at the end of this book in the *Making Oils* chapter.

One more valuable burn remedy for the first aid kit is **vitamin E** oil. A bottle of the oil is most convenient, but capsules can be used as long as you have easy access to a puncture tool. Toothpicks work well for puncturing a vitamin E capsule, and they store easily in your kit. Always make sure the oil you use is naturally derived and not synthetic vitamin E.

Find it Fast

1st **Degree:** Symptoms include red skin, often some swelling, and sometimes pain. Wash well with cool water for several minutes. Apply cool wet compresses or a fresh aloe leaf (sliced lengthwise to expose gel) for 10 to 30 minutes. Gently pat dry and apply more gel. Do not cover burn with bandages; exposure to air will hasten healing. Calendula oil and/or aloe vera gel can be reapplied as needed over the following days.

2nd **Degree:** Symptoms include blisters and very red and blotchy skin with severe pain and swelling. Treat as you would a 1st degree burn. Including vitamin E oil as a follow-up treatment is helpful for a more severe burn. Do NOT break skin blisters, as this increases the risk of infection. Calendula oil, aloe vera gel, and/or vitamin E oil can be reapplied as needed over the following days.

3rd **Degree:** Symptoms include burning through all skin layers, often resulting in a black or charred appearance, or even dry and white skin. If it's a small burn and not on delicate skin, you can treat it the same as you would a 2nd degree burn, followed by an immediate trip to the doctor. If it's a larger burn or in a sensitive area, seek emergency treatment immediately. Do not attempt to remove any clothing touching the area. Don't immerse large 3rd degree burns in cold water. Elevate the burned body part if possible. If breathing has stopped, start CPR immediately.

In the days that follow emergency treatment, calendula oil, aloe vera gel, and/or vitamin E oil can be reapplied as needed as permitted by your doctor.

When to Call 9-1-1

When any one of the following symptoms are present, call 9-1-1 or your local emergency number:

- Trouble breathing.
- Burns that either cover more than one part of the body or burns that cover a large area.
- Burns on the head, neck, feet, hands, or genitals.
- Burns involving the mouth or nose, or burns that somehow restrict breathing.
- Burns caused by explosion, electricity, or chemicals.
- Deeply penetrating burns of any size, especially in children under the age of five years and adults over the age of 60.

Chest Pains

The statistics aren't pleasant: About 900,000 people die from some form of heart disease each year in the U.S. alone. It is the number one cause of death in this country. For a young person in good health, this could seem like an easy statistic to ignore, but even if you and your husband are youthful marathon runners with young children, don't make the mistake of thinking heart attack preparedness is for your grandma's kit alone. Keep these remedies on hand and know what to do in an emergency. If not for your young and healthy family, then for a visiting friend or family member who may need you.

Chest Pain Remedies

Let me start by saying that if there is a heart patient in your home, you should keep nitroglycerin tablets or other prescribed emergency medication in your first aid kit at all times, as well as being carried on that person. If you or someone else is experiencing heart attack symptoms, call 9-1-1 immediately. According to the American Red Cross, over half of all heart attack victims wait over two hours to call for help. This is way too long to wait. See the Find it Fast section below for a full list of common symptoms.

While there isn't an herbal remedy that magically stops a heart attack, there are herbal remedies that can assist with chest pains caused by a myriad of issues, even stepping in when nitroglycerin tablets or other heart medications aren't available to you. One such herbal powerhouse is hawthorn.

Hawthorn (*Crataegus spp.*) is THE heart health tonic herb. I'm not alone in saying that. Herbalists the world over recommend hawthorn for numerous heart issues. If taken regularly, it has the ability to strengthen overall heart health and improve circulation. Its dilating power improves blood flow and can bring relief when there's a more minor coronary incident, like when your heart skips a beat or there's an unusual flutter. While hawthorn is usually considered too slow to replace nitro tablets, hawthorn is used in Germany to treat milder cases of heart failure. If you get heart palpitations from lying down or sitting, or if you skip a beat when you inhale, hawthorn can adjust it.

Adding **passionflower** (*Passiflora caerulea* or *incarnata*) to your kit will provide extra heart protection. It's effective immediately when nitroglycerin or other medications are not available. It relaxes the arteries and works well with hawthorn. As an arterial sedative, it can even out some of those heart irregularities.

Find it Fast

Heart Irregularities/Chest Pain: Administer hawthorn tincture or a combination of hawthorn and passionflower tinctures. Take 10 to 30 drops of hawthorn and/or 20 to 40 drops of passionflower tinctures in water.

Heart Attack: If nitroglycerin tablets or other emergency medications are not available, administer hawthorn and/or passionflower tinctures and call 9-1-1 immediately. Take 10 to 30 drops of hawthorn and/or 20 to 40 drops of passionflower tinctures in water.

When to Call 9-1-1

When any of the following symptoms are present, call 9-1-1 or your local emergency number immediately:

- Chest pain that lasts longer than three to five minutes, or if it goes away and comes back. (This is usually described as a presence of tightness, pressure, achiness, squeezing, or a sense of heaviness. Brief and stabbing pain that increases when you bend over or breathe deeply is not usually a sign of heart problems.)

- Chest pain that spreads to the shoulder, arm, neck, stomach, or back.

Other Signs of a Heart Attack

The pain of a heart attack varies from discomfort to unbearable and crushing pain. Many times an attack starts out slowly and builds, the pain being felt in the center of the chest. Also look for shortness of breath, pale or gray skin, sensations of dizziness or nausea, heavy sweating, and/or fatigue. Signs for men and women are largely the same, but women tend toward more shortness of breath, nausea, and vomiting. They may also feel the pain in the back or in the jaw, and may experience malaise. The pain experienced by women is oftentimes sharp and sudden.

Ear Infections

Ear infections are increasingly more common among children. Reasons vary, including a cold or flu virus; food allergies or improper diet; and bottle feeding while in repose, resulting in moisture buildup in the ear canal. But no matter the cause, an ear infection is horribly painful for any age. Most infections don't result in a trip to the emergency room or the doctor's office, and will clear up on their own if taken care of properly. But ask any child and they'll tell you; the pain feels like a definite emergency. Let's include a few natural remedies to ease the pain and perhaps clear things up enough that visiting the doctor is no longer necessary.

Ear Remedies

It's important to keep a small bottle of **hydrogen peroxide** in your kit, and here's one good reason why: Ear infections are often seated deep in the canal, but a few drops of peroxide in the infected ear can help turn things around.

St. John's-wort (*Hypericum perforatum*) oil is hands down my favorite remedy for ear pain. I am never without a bottle of the oil because its pain relieving power is incredible, especially for sensitive and painful ears. Even deep down pain can be relieved with a minimal application of oil, and fast. My own experience is that even severe pain is gone in anywhere from 15 seconds to a minute if the oil is of good quality. It's best if you can make your own, but it's not practical for most people. St. John's-wort oil is available at health food stores and online and is worth the effort to find it. If you want to go the extra mile, instructions for making your own can be found in the *Making Oils* chapter of this book.

If the peroxide fizzed a lot while in the ear canal, that's a good indication that there is infection present, and that the peroxide is dealing with it. Using your **echinacea** (*Echinacea purpurea* or *angustifolia*) tincture will also help you fight it off. Be sure to adjust the diet and stay away from processed sugar, juice, and yeast products until the infection has completely cleared.

Find it Fast

Hydrogen Peroxide: Using an eye dropper, place just two or three drops in the infected ear while the head is tipped. This will allow the peroxide to go into the ear without running back out. Once the fizzing has stopped, tip the head to release the peroxide onto a towel or cotton ball.

St. John's-wort Oil: Using an eye dropper, place one or two drops of oil in the infected ear while the head is tipped. Stay still for a few minutes to allow the oil to work its way in. If desired, place a cotton ball in the opening of the ear to keep the oil from dripping back out. Alternatively, the oil can be placed into the outer part of the ear canal using a cotton swab. Even if the ear pain is deep, this is often enough to relieve it.

Echinacea Tincture: At the first signs of infection, take 30 to 100 drops of tincture in a bit of water. Repeat every one to two hours until symptoms start to subside. Continue taking 20 to 30 drops of tincture in water up to five times a day until the infection is completely gone.

When to See a Doctor

- Severe pain.

- Symptoms that last more than a day.

- Blood, pus, or fluid drainage from the ear canal.

Eye Conditions

Few stories exemplify my lack of grace and aptitude in sports such as this one. I was twelve and my sister was nine. My parents had put up an old badminton set in the backyard, and I was taking my role as older sister seriously, instructing her on the finer points of serving the birdie. We worked and worked at it, and eventually she was getting the hang of swinging the racket. So I moved back to my side of the net and hit a nice gentle serve. My sister, who has always had more athletic prowess than I, wound up and really let that poor birdie have it. It cleared the net with great force and whacked me in the eye.

I was later told that her serve had so much gusto that it knocked me to my knees. I just remember not seeing anything. At all. My pupil looked like nothing more than a tiny pinprick, and by the time the intense white light faded away and I realized I had not actually died, my mom already had us loaded up in the van and halfway to the emergency room.

Fortunately, it was nothing more than a minor scratch, but

the doctors insisted I wear a big patch over my eye every day for a week, which really cramped my sixth grade style. The big hunk of gauze clashed with my Dorothy Hamill glasses, and we won't even mention the night brace my orthodontist decided must be worn all day.

It was my prime ugly duckling moment. I have a feeling that a few herbal remedies could have sped up the process, maybe helped me ditch the eye patch sooner. No amount of herbs could have melted the Hamill glasses, but at least I would have been as bi-orbital as my classmates.

Eye Remedies

Perhaps you think its main benefit is inducing sleep, but **chamomile** (*Matricaria recutita*) has a list of medicinal uses that far exceeds most people's expectations. As a tea, it is a helpful eyewash for everything from conjunctivitis (pink eye) and minor scratches to irritated and bloodshot eyes. It's a soothing and natural anti-inflammatory, and you can even use it in a cool compress if you happen to get a badminton-type bonk.

A **golden seal** (*Hydrastis canadensis*) wash is another

effective treatment for conjunctivitis and otherwise itchy, irritated eyes. Using just a few drops of golden seal tincture in some isotonic water will provide a healing eyewash.

If you get a liquid irritant splashed in the eye, such as a chemical household cleaner, you should flush your eye out in the sink with water immediately. If the eye burns or stings, have someone call emergency as you continue to wash out the eye. Be sure to tilt your head in the sink so that the affected eye is the one lower than the healthy eye, so you don't accidentally rinse the irritant from one side into the other.

Probably the most interesting eye remedy you'll ever hear is one I learned of from a Native American herbalism class. An old Chumash remedy, the Southwest Native Americans relied on the tiny **chia** seed (*Salvia hispanica*) to remove pesky little irritants from the eye. Chia, the seed more popularly known as part of a kitchy Christmas gift that grows green hair on terra cotta bulls and cats, really comes from a sage plant. It excels at growing in areas that recently suffered a wildfire. Just one tiny drop of water and the seed grows a gelatinous coating that sucks up and holds onto the moisture, thus helping a seed to germinate under the driest of conditions.

To use the chia as a remedy requires the presoaking of a single little seed. The seed, now soft and squishy, can be placed beneath the lower lid of the eye overnight, where it attracts any tiny particles or bits of dust and foreign matter that may be the cause of your irritation. The seed is perfectly comfortable there, and you'll never notice it. During the night it will also sooth the eye membrane. In the morning, remove the seed carefully with clean hands.

Find it Fast

Chemical/Harmful Liquid Splash: Immediately begin flushing out the eye with water, being sure to keep the head tipped in the sink in such a way that the affected eye is below the healthy eye. Have someone call 9-1-1 and don't stop rinsing out the eye until help arrives.

Conjunctivitis: Prepare a cup of chamomile tea by steeping one teaspoon of herb in one cup of hot water for 15 to 20 minutes. Strain well and wait for the tea to cool. Leaning over the sink, slowly pour the tea over the eye. Repeat this process several times a day until the infection clears. Or use five drops of golden seal tincture per tablespoon of isotonic water and, using an eyedropper, place a few drops in the eye. Repeat several times a day until the infection clears.

Minor Scratches/Bloodshot Eyes: Prepare chamomile tea and use as a wash, as instructed above. You can also dip a clean cloth in the cooled tea to be used as a compress.

Foreign Object/Dust: If the foreign object is lodged into the eyeball, do NOT attempt to remove it yourself. Call 9-1-1 and wait for emergency help. If the object is very small such as dust or a minute particle that's causing mild irritation, soak one chia seed in water for 10 minutes. Place the single seed under the bottom eyelid and leave it there for several hours. This remedy works best when used overnight. In the morning, remove the seed carefully with clean hands.

When to Call 9-1-1

- Serious pain and/or bleeding is present.
- Foreign object stuck into the eye, such as a splinter.
- Chemicals or other dangerous liquid splashed in the eyes.

Fevers

You kept your child home from school today. She's acting just fine and has even been racing around the house, much to your astonishment; her high fever and runny nose don't seem to slow her down. Unfortunately, you don't have the energy to keep up with her because you have the same high fever and runny nose. But you don't feel the least bit like playing "chase the mommy" with her. You're more concerned with keeping yourself upright.

Fevers sometimes have a way of leveling adults while leaving kids with enough energy to overtake a small country. But no matter the age, a persistently high fever can usually be broken with the right herbal remedy.

Fever Remedies

It's important to know what's causing a fever before attempting to break it. Not every fever is meant to be broken, after all. If you've had a virus for a couple of days and the fever is high but not over 103 F (39.4 C), breaking a fever is fine. Anything higher should not be broken but should be cared for by a doctor. The process of breaking a fever temporarily spikes it a bit higher, so if you already have a very high fever, don't attempt these remedies.

Ginger (*Zingiber officinalis*) tea is one of the more pleasant ways to break the fever. The tea can be prepared from either dried root or fresh, and the warm, spicy flavor can be enhanced with some honey for a delicious tea that also helps calm stomachs, ease headaches, and relieve the other aches and pains that you might experience with a virus.

Boneset (*Eupatorium perfoliatum*) is an effective fever reducer and is my preferred choice when the fever comes from a cold, flu, or viral infection. It's also an immune stimulant and pain reducer specializing in achy bones, so it should play a hefty role in your herbal arsenal during cold and flu season.

Find it Fast

Ginger: Steep one teaspoon of dried ginger in a cup of hot water for 15 to 20 minutes. Sweeten with honey if you prefer. Drink as needed.

Boneset: Twenty to 40 drops of tincture in hot water, taken up to three times daily.

When to Call 9-1-1

Call for emergency help if a high fever is paired with a combination of any of these symptoms:

- Severe headache
- Persistent vomiting
- Breathing difficulties
- Chest pain
- Unusual rash
- Eyes unusually sensitive to bright light
- Stiff neck
- Pain felt when head is tipped forward
- Extreme irritability or listlessness
- Severe abdominal pain or pain during urination
- Mental confusion

You should seek medical help in the following instances:

- Baby under three months with a rectal temperature of 100.4 F (38 C) or higher, even if no other symptoms exist.

- Baby older than three months has temperature of 102 F (38.9 C) or higher.

- Child under the age of two with fever for longer than one day; child two years or older with a fever lasting longer than three days.

- Adult with temperature of 103 F (39.4 C) or has had any fever for more than three days.

Heatstroke & Overheating

Grandma's been sick lately; she's convalescing after a long hospital stay. You've got a good heart, so you packed her up with the family and took her to a day at the lake. You took the sun umbrella, ice water, even a great big sun hat you thought Granny would appreciate. She wore it for exactly three minutes before tossing it aside, claiming it made her head itch. The umbrella cast too dark a shadow on her issue of Woman's Day, so she sat in the direct sun for most of the afternoon. Ice water? No thanks. She claims a sore throat and gives you that look that says, "Leave me alone. I remember you in diapers." She was stubborn enough to find her way to heatstroke, despite all your best efforts. But you've got your first aid kit stashed in the car. Because this isn't the first time Granny's pulled this one on you.

Heatstroke & Overheating Remedies

It's important to determine whether or not Grandma's just overheated from too much sun or if she is indeed having heatstroke. Heatstroke is considered an emergency situation and requires immediate emergency attention. So look for signals such as dizziness, headaches, nausea, high body temperature, even staggering. Those who are in poor health, are alcoholics over the age of 40, or are overtired before being exposed to high heat are more likely to get heatstroke than healthy individuals.

The remedies for heatstroke and overheating are neat and tidy. **Lemon balm** (*Melissa officinalis*) tincture is both relaxing and cooling to the system and is pleasant to take. It's a mild sedative that won't knock you out, and its anti-inflammatory properties will help work on that headache while regulating your internal temperature. Alternatively, the dried herbs make a wonderful tea that's nice served cold.

Angelica (*Angelica archangelica*) seeds store well in a kit and require only that you chew a few to cool off. They also double as a stomach aid; cramping, indigestion, colic, and flatulence can also be relieved with these tiny little seeds.

Hibiscus (*Hibiscus sabdariffa*) tea both cools and lowers blood pressure. The tea is a beautiful ruby red color that has the tang of citrus. Served hot or cold, it's excellent. My favorite way to prepare it is as a sun tea, but that's for pleasure. In an emergency, the hot tea is much quicker.

While you can't store fresh food in your kit, you can rely on things such as cucumber or watermelon to turn heatstroke around. These foods, along with any citrus, have amazing cooling properties. So if you're packing Granny up for another beach trip, be sure to take a nice cucumber salad and a watermelon along.

Find it Fast

Heatstroke: Call 9-1-1 immediately. Get the person out of the heat and sun, and if possible, give them a cold bath or shower until help arrives. Hibiscus tea can be used while waiting for the ambulance. Do NOT allow the person to fall asleep.

Overheating: Take 20 to 40 drops of lemon balm tincture in a small amount of water as needed. Or prepare one teaspoon dried (but not old) herb in one cup hot water. Steep for 15 to 20 minutes. Drink as needed. Prepare hibiscus tea in the same way. Serve either one hot or cold. One to two angelica seeds can also be chewed as needed.

When to Call 9-1-1
- Feeling weak, dizzy, or tired.
- Headaches and/or seeing spots.
- Nausea.
- Loss of appetite.
- Ringing ears.
- Red skin and/or elevated body temperature.
- Difficulty breathing.
- Staggering or difficulty walking.

Nausea & Vomiting

Let's see a show of hands: Who likes to vomit?

Just as I suspected. There's only one of you with his hand up, and he's way in the back of the room, looking a bit off.

There are some very effective herbal remedies for putting a quick stop to nausea and vomiting without knocking you out or having to endure drinking any pink goop. They'll be easy to store in your first aid kit, and they taste better, too. Whether the issue is motion sickness, stomach flu, or a bad pot sticker, there's an herb to rescue you.

Nausea & Vomiting Remedies

Cardamom (*Elettaria cardamomum*) pods are the perfect prepackaged nausea and motion sickness remedy. Inexpensive if purchased in bulk in most cooking stores, the pods can be kept for several years in a small tin in your first aid kit and still be ready to assist you. Peel away the hull and remove one or two little black seeds and chew or suck on them for relief from nausea, queasiness, and vomiting. This is also a safe one for expectant mothers who are experiencing morning sickness.

For both diarrhea and vomiting, **peppermint** (Mentha piperita) could be nicknamed "Old Reliable." A mug of the tea is often enough to turn things around and settle many digestive complaints, and it's safe for all ages. Another alternative is **catmint** (*Nepeta cataria*) which plays double duty by soothing the stomach and relaxing the individual, enough to sleep soundly without a druggy feeling. It also relaxes stomach cramps and is good for everyone from baby to Grandma.

Let's not forget **chamomile** (*Matricaria recutita*) It's going to be an important part of your first aid kit, so stock up on it. Relaxing to both spirit and body, chamomile turns around upset stomachs, vomiting, and diarrhea. Again, it's appropriate for any age.

Find it Fast

Cardamom Pods: Peel hull from one pod and suck on or chew one to two seeds. Seeds can then be discarded or swallowed after use. Repeat as needed.

Peppermint: Steep one teaspoon of the dried herb in one cup of water for 15 to 20 minutes. Drink as needed.

Catmint: Steep one teaspoon of the dried herb in one cup of water for 15 to 20 minutes. Drink as needed.

When to Call 9-1-1

- Chest pain is also present.
- Severe abdominal pain or cramping.
- Fainting.
- Loss of consciousness.
- Confusion.
- Pale skin that is cold or clammy to the touch.
- High fever coupled with a stiff neck.
- Blood or fecal matter and/or fecal odor in the vomit.
- Severe headache, especially if it's the sort of

headache you've not experienced previously.

- For adults: Unable to eat or drink anything in the past 12 hours. For children: Unable to keep liquids down in the past 8 hours.

- Vomit resembles coffee grounds or is green.

Pain Relief

No matter the emergency, pain is more than likely involved. No first aid kit would be complete without a good set of pain relievers, and there are several herbal remedies to choose from in this instance. In my experience, the following are some of the best and can easily outdo the most popular over-the-counter medications. Any good owl will tell you to package them up in smaller amounts for your kit and keep the rest in your medicine cabinet for the everyday aches and pains.

Pain Remedies

Aspirin is not an anti-inflammatory, but its original and natural source is. **Willow bark** (*Salix spp.*) contains salicin and is nature's true aspirin. It's an all-purpose pain reliever for everything from arthritis to headaches (especially feverish ones), sore muscles to urethritis. You can even gargle with the tea for relief of a sore throat.

If you're prone to migraines, you should probably keep some **feverfew** (*Chrysanthemum parthenium*) stocked up. While the tea is effective, the tincture doesn't need to steep, thus it provides faster relief - an important consideration, as any migraine sufferer will tell you. Another great anti-inflammatory, feverfew will also help rid you of menstrual cramps, stomachaches, toothaches, and general aches and pains.

When pain is severe such as with a broken bone, torn ligament, or strained back, you can rely on **valerian** (*Valeriana spp.*) to ease even the toughest of aches. Since valium gets its pain busting power from valerian, you can go straight to the herbal source and skip the side effects. Valerian is for big pain that causes restlessness and sleeplessness. This is too strong for kids (ironically, it often winds them up) but adults will appreciate the knock-out effect it has, giving someone a deep and painless sleep that is often just what's needed for quicker healing.

A nerve sedative will prove a good addition to your first aid tools. **St. John's-wort** (*Hypericum perforatum*) oil can be applied topically to calm noisy nerves and is a good choice for nighttime irritations that won't let you sleep.

Find it Fast

Willow Bark: General pain relief, anti-inflammatory. Mix one teaspoon of dried herb in 1 ½ cups of water and simmer for 20 to 30 minutes. Strain. Drink two to four ounces up to four times daily.

Feverfew: General pain relief, anti-inflammatory. If using tincture, take 30 to 60 drops in a small amount of water up to four times a day. If tea is preferred, steep one teaspoon in hot water for 15 to 20 minutes. Drink as needed.

Valerian: Severe pain resulting in sleeplessness. Take 30 to 90 drops of tincture in some water up to three times daily. Or steep one teaspoon of dried herb in one cup of very hot water for 15 to 20 minutes. Drink four to six ounces up to three times daily. **NOTE**: Valerian is not for regular use and should not be taken for more than a few weeks at a time. Some people do experience a sense of agitation while taking valerian; if this is you, discontinue use. Not for children.

St. John's-wort Oil: Nerve sedative. Apply oil to the irritated nerve pathway; for instance, if a pinched nerve occurs in the back, find that area and apply topically. Use as needed.

When to See a Doctor

- Any persistent or severe pain, especially pain that does not go away shortly, should be checked out by a doctor.

Poisonous Plants

That wasn't a grapevine he was climbing. Your son realizes it now, but it's too late for his newfound knowledge to help him out of it. He's covered in a red rash from head to foot. Who knew he was such a thorough climber? Your mother used to blot you in pink dots of calamine lotion when you got in similar scrapes, and while it did bring you relief, you didn't appreciate looking like something from a Willy Wonka movie. Your son is even less likely to appreciate that particular shade of glowing pink. What's a natural mom to do? Hand him a bamboo back scratcher? No, you've got herbs for this.

Poisonous Plant Remedies

For the most part, the effects of poison ivy, poison oak, and poison sumac take time to get over, with or without the remedies. But when it comes to combating itchy, scratchy plant reactions, **jewelweed** (*Impatiens capensis*) is the winner in the herb world. Ironically, it likes to grow in areas where poison ivy is present. The beautiful little orange flowers look like charming fairy hats, and the ripe seed pods literally explode when touched, giving them the common name "touch-me-not". While jewelweed does its best work when used fresh, not many people have access to it. And even if it does grow in your yard, it won't work unless it's in flower. But the good news here is that jewelweed soap is available ready made. You can pick up a bar from various home and garden stores, health food stores such as Whole Foods, even Etsy. Prices range from $4 to $10 for a bar. It should be included in your first aid kit.

If you're feeling especially industrious and you know how to identify jewelweed, you can harvest the flowers from early summer until the first frost and prepare your own salve to keep until you need it. (See the *Making Salves* chapter of this book for instructions.)

Echinacea (*Echinacea angustifolia* or *purpurea*) enters the picture once again, proving its usefulness as part of your natural first aid kit. The tincture can be applied topically, as can **elder flower** (*Sambucus nigra*) tea. But in the end, the most reliable remedy for poison ivy, oak, and sumac rashes is jewelweed.

Find it Fast

Jewelweed: If using soap, follow the soapmaker's instructions. If using salve, apply liberally to clean dry skin; use as needed.

Echinacea: Apply tincture externally. If tincture stings, squirt a few droppersful in some warm water and apply as needed.

Elder Flower: Steep one teaspoon of dried elder flowers in a cup of hot water for 15 to 20 minutes. Strain and apply topically when cool. Repeat as needed.

Weeping Sores: If weeping sores are present, apply elder flower tea or prepare a paste of baking soda and water. Apply topically as needed.

When to See a Doctor
- Reaction appears severe or covers much of the body.
- The rash has spread to face and/or genitals.
- Fever over 100 F (37.8 C).
- Pus-filled blisters present.
- Rash that lasts more than a few weeks.

Strains & Sprains

You woke up with a wild hair and decided to give the basement a thorough cleaning, and without anyone's help. Everything was going according to plan until you picked up that old computer monitor all by yourself - or should I say "tried to"? You knew you were in trouble as soon as that familiar tug occurred at the base of your spine. You also knew you wouldn't be moving from that spot of the furnace room anytime soon. If your daughter hadn't come downstairs when she did, it's possible no one would have discovered you were missing until they got hungry for dinner.

Strain & Sprain Remedies

You can't underestimate the power of a simple **ice pack** for the pull of a back or the twist of an ankle. Whether it's a first aid ice pack stored in the freezer, the disposable instant cold compresses included in most premade first aid kits, or a basic bag of frozen peas, applying cold to the injury will help reduce both the swelling and the pain.

St. John's-wort oil (*Hypericum perforatum*) can be applied topically for a strain or a sprain, which will relieve the pain, reducing the swelling and inflammation, and lessen any bruising that may occur. This is a good follow-up remedy to use after you've iced your injury.

If the pain is just too much after icing your sprain, you can take **valerian** (*Valeriana spp.*) for some rest and relief. While this tincture isn't the pain reliever you'd want to take for minor pains or aches, it's an excellent choice for adults. (Not suitable for children.)

*See the *Pain Relief* chapter of this book for more options.

Toothaches

Cavities, broken teeth, root canals: words that can make anyone cringe in remembrance. While you can't fill a cavity with a poultice, and it isn't possible to perform a root canal using a pointy dandelion leaf, you can stave off the pain until you get to the dentist, and you can certainly curb the discomfort that results from visiting him. Remember not to forget the remedies available in the *Pain Relief* chapter, either. You can use them in combination with the following tips for the safe and natural alleviation of your tooth woes.

Toothache Remedies

The herb **feverfew** (*Chrysanthemum parthenium*) isn't just for migraines. It's able to curb the pain of many a toothache as well. Drink the tea, rinse out your mouth with it, or use the tincture in a bit of warm water for similar fast acting results.

An old time remedy your mother may have used on your gums back when you were teething, **clove** (*Syzygium aromaticum*) oil is still a preferred option for teething and tooth pain. The essential oil will keep well in your kit, and when applied topically, it knocks out the pain in a hurry. And let's not forget the resulting breath will be fresh and spicy.

Keeping a small packet of **sea salt** in your kit for the occasional toothache is a good idea. Mixing it with some warm water gives a nice mouth rinse that can be used to clean the affected area while neutralizing the pain. You can then follow up with the clove oil, if you wish.

Find it Fast

Feverfew: Steep one teaspoon of dried herb in one cup of hot water for 15 to 20 minutes. Use the warm tea as a mouth rinse and/or drink two to four ounces, up to four times daily, for pain relief.

Clove Oil: Using a pure essential oil and not a blend or a flavoring used for baking, apply a drop or two of oil to the affected area using a cotton swab or cotton ball. If using on babies or young children, apply a minimal amount; this remedy can become a bit too spicy for younger palates.

Sea Salt: Dissolve one teaspoon of sea salt in eight ounces of warm water. Swish the solution in the mouth for about one minute, then spit. Repeat as necessary. This is a good technique to use before applying the clove oil.

When to See Your Dentist

- Experiencing any tooth pain at all is reason to visit your dentist. Using remedies to curtail pain associated with cavities, abscesses, or any other tooth issues should be viewed as a temporary measure until proper dental attention can be had.

Wounds

There's a good chance the most action your first aid kit will see will be for the treatment of cuts and wounds, especially if you have any children. Whether your child is learning to ride a bike, climb a tree, or even walk for the first time, bumps and bruises will most likely accompany these milestones on occasion. But you'll be prepared with a few easy and essential first aid herbal remedies. Don't forget that magic kiss to make it all better. (Sock puppets and teddy bears are also a nice touch.)

Wound Remedies

Salves, tinctures, and teas all play an important part in treating cuts and wounds with herbs. But first, washing the wound with soap and water is key. Some of these herbal remedies can work fast, sealing in any dirt or foreign matter. So make sure to flush the wound thoroughly under running water.

To build up bacterial resistance, **echinacea** (*Echinacea angustifolia* or *purpurea*) is a wonderful tincture that can reduce the chances of septicemia setting in. The tincture can be used both externally and internally. After washing a wound, a few drops of tincture can be applied. A parental warning: This will sting. Tinctures contain alcohol, so if the cut is deep or the child is sensitive, you can instead offer some tincture to drink in a little water or juice. The benefits are the same, if only slightly delayed.

Golden seal (*Hydrastis canadensis*) tincture can be applied topically to a wound of any sort. It's a great antimicrobial that won't shrink or tan the skin, and it won't create an isolated pus pocket. That's because it promotes healing from the inside out, rather than growing the skin over the wound before internal healing can happen. (Still be sure to wash the area thoroughly before application.) Again, applying the tincture to an open sore will sting, but it's beneficial topically. For more sensitive people, try putting a few drops of the tincture into some water and rinsing the wound, rather than going with a straight shot.

Calendula (*Calendula officinalis*) is antibacterial, antiviral, and anti-inflammatory. I can't imagine building an herbal first aid kit without it. If the injury is deep or severe, use it as a follow-up treatment to prevent infection and to greatly reduce or eliminate the possibility of a scar. It promotes healing and can hasten the growth of new and healthy skin. It even reduces pain, so it's an all-in-one herbal healer.

While a tea of calendula can be applied topically, I prefer a salve preparation. This does require more effort than just putting a container of dried flowers in the kit, however, but it's worth it. Complete instructions for calendula salve can be found in the Making Salves portion of the book.

For minor skin abrasions and bruises, a gentle tea of **hyssop** (*Hyssopus officinalis*) can be applied topically. It's antiviral and anti-inflammatory, and it's able to cope with the strained muscles that may have occurred due to the stress of a fall or accident. If the incident caused any anxiety, have a cup to drink, and enjoy its relaxing properties. The perfect choice for children as well as adults.

Bleeding can be stopped in a hurry with one of my favorite first aid remedies: **yarrow** (*Achillea millefolium*). Whether you choose tea, tincture, or a poultice of fresh leaves, you've got a mighty powerful hemostatic. I used this on a deep cut on my thumb once after lancing it open with a gardening tool while harvesting yarrow. (The irony hurts, doesn't it?) The cut was sealed within a minute or two of holding chewed yarrow leaves on the cut. While I wouldn't recommend chewing the leaves first, it does work if you've no mortar and pestle about, and if the cut needs immediate closure as mine did. Otherwise, rinsing with the tea or applying the tincture will produce fast healing, although for ease of use and storage, I prefer yarrow salve. It keeps well, doesn't sting, and you don't have to wait for a tea to steep. (Instructions for preparation are in the *Making Salve* chapter of this book.)

Making Medicinal Oils & Salves

Although making your own medicinal oils and salves for your first aid kit isn't a necessary task, it is fun, easy, and cost effective. These oils and salves are available commercially, but if you feel like tapping into your pioneer spirit, give the following recipes a whirl.

St. John's-wort and calendula are the oils I recommend having for your kit. The others mentioned in this chapter - plantain, jewelweed, and yarrow - are oils that you'll need to prepare if you decide to make your own salves. These salves can also be purchased in many health food stores or online, if you'd prefer not to make your own.

While dried plants can often be used, all of these oils work best if prepared with fresh plants; but it's especially important if you're making St. John's-wort or jewelweed oil. In the case of St. John's-wort and jewelweed, the oils just don't come out very nicely using the dried plants, as drying them causes the loss of many of the constituents that give the plants their effectiveness. If you're going to prepare an oil from fresh flowers and leaves, you'll have to do a bit of wildcrafting unless you're lucky enough to have these

75

growing in your garden. If you don't know how to identify these plants already, get a good field guide for your area of the country or world, and check out websites such as www.eol.org where lots of good photography exists. Only one of these plants can be harvested year round: plantain. Even digging it up from the snow is acceptable. I do prefer a nice spring plantain, but I've used it in all seasons, and it does indeed work. The others are summer plants.

If you've decided to make your oil using dried herb, you've got one thing going for you: The plants are available year round. No waiting around for them to come into bloom or for the snow to melt.

What You'll Need:

A medium saucepan
Glass measuring cup, 2-cup size
Sweet almond oil (food grade) or olive oil
Clean dry jars with tight-fitting lids for the oils
Enough fresh flowers or leaves, or ground dried herbs, to fill a jar when loosely packed
A chopstick or other stick-type pokey thing to knock out air bubbles

If Making Salve from the Oil:

Beeswax (Pastilles or grated are easiest to work with.)

Natural vitamin E gel capsules

Tins or other containers, preferably opaque

If using freshly picked plant material, shake off any debris and remove any dead or unhealthy looking leaves or flowers. Chop the fresh herbs or grind the dried herbs, then fill your jar with the plants and push them down gently. You want plenty in the jar, but it shouldn't be so tightly packed that oil will not be able to penetrate it.

Now fill the jar to the top with oil. Either olive oil or sweet almond oil are good choices, as both have a longer shelf life and are capable of delivering the medicinal properties deep into the skin. Sweet almond oil has no fragrance to speak of, but olive oil will leave a bit of its scent behind, so if you don't care for an olive oil fragrance, sweet almond is the better choice.

Using your wooden chopstick or other pokey device, push the plant material down into the jar so as to release as much of the trapped air as possible. This will help keep the oil from going rancid. Now cap the jar and make sure it's a tight seal. If it isn't tight enough for comfort, wrap a bit of plastic wrap over the top of the open jar, then cap it tightly. This is usually enough to create a tighter seal.

If you're still concerned about air bubbles, you can lightly thunk the jar on a tabletop a few times. (I once met an herbalist who liked to carry his steeping oil in his car, then drive back and forth on the dirt road in front of his house. Perhaps one could say that's taking it a bit too far, but I'd do that in a heartbeat if my street wasn't paved.)

Now place the jar in a sunny window and allow it to steep for a solid two weeks before using it. Don't shake it; just leave it to do its thing. If you're making St. John's-wort oil, you'll notice it will turn a lovely shade that ranges somewhere between a deep orangey red and a ruby red color; the prettiest of the oils, in my opinion.

When the time is up, dump the entire contents of the jar, oil and all, into the large glass measuring cup. Take a paper towel and fold it into fourths, placing it in the bottom of your pan. This gives a bit of a safety buffer between the glass cup and the hot metal pan. Add enough water to the pan (NOT the measuring cup) so that the level of the water is equal to or above that of the oil in the cup.

Turn the heat on very, very low. Do NOT allow the water to boil, as this will destroy the medicinal properties. The point here is to slowly steep the herbs in the oil. Allow them to steep for about 30 minutes, paying special attention to your water level. It should at all times remain equal to or above the oil.

Once your timer has alerted you to the end of your waiting, you can turn off the heat and allow the oil to fully cool. Strain the oil through an old wire mesh colander, squeezing the plant material with clean hands to remove as much of the oil as possible.

If the oil you've just prepared is to remain a medicinal oil and was not made for use in a salve, you can now pour the oil into jars and cap tightly. Label the jars with a date and the name of the herb, and be sure to store some in your first aid kit. Any remaining oil should be stored in a dark place, somewhere out of extreme temperature changes.

If you plan to prepare a salve with your oil, pour the oil back into the measuring cup and put the cup back into the pan. Now add the beeswax.

To determine how much beeswax should be used, figure on adding ⅙ the amount of oil you have. So if you have one full cup of oil, you'll need to add ⅙ a cup of beeswax.

Top up the water level in the pan, if needed. Turn the heat back on very low, and heat until all the beeswax has melted. Sometimes it's helpful if you poke at it with that pokey tool you used earlier. Stirring helps too, and although I've never seen it do any good, talking to it at least passes the time until it all decides to melt.

When the last bit of beeswax has melted, take a small spoonful of the mixture and put it on a small plate for testing. Put the plate in the freezer for a minute to allow it to fully cool, then take it out and examine the consistency. Salve should be thick but not solid; it needs to be smooth enough to rub into the skin, yet still hold together nicely in the container. If your salve seems too sloppy for you, add a bit more beeswax to the mixture in the pan and continue to heat until it melts. Repeat the testing until the consistency is where you like it.

Turn off the heat and squeeze in the contents of a couple of vitamin E capsules, about one capsule per every four ounces of salve.

Now pour your liquefied salve into the salve containers and leave the containers uncapped until the salve is completely cooled. Cap and label the containers with the date and the salve type. Be sure to add one container of each salve variety to your kit, then store any remaining tins or containers out of direct sunlight and extreme heat or cold.

Making Tinctures

One of my favorite activities in herbalism is making tincture. There's something neat and tidy about it on the one hand, and something wild and messy about it on the other, that really appeals to both sides of my split personality. I can enjoy the messiness of wildcrafting herbs from the forest; the hunt for a stand of a long searched-for herb, the dirt under my nails, the smell of the herbs when they're picked, a connection to nature. Then when I get them back home, I can examine them like the mad scientist I wish I were, holding them up to the light and picking off any tiny imperfections and covering them with alcohol in clear glass jars, which I then line up on my shelves.

The first time I ever made a tincture, I felt intimidated by the process. This was real herbal medicine, and I was about to make some. But after that first jar was complete, it was beautiful and it connected me to both nature and the past in a way I didn't expect. And it was easier than I'd thought. Now, my shelves are lined with jar after jar of sparkling tinctures.

The tinctures recommended for your first aid kit are the following: Echinacea, hawthorn, passionflower, golden seal, lemon balm, valerian, and yarrow. Of course, you can go to the health food store or hop online and buy any or all of these, but if you can, try to make at least one of these tinctures on your own.

Tinctures can be made from dried or fresh herbs, and while I definitely prefer fresh, it's not always available. Echinacea, for instance, is a protected plant in the United States, so unless you grow your own, purchasing ethically harvested dried root is probably your best bet. (Occasionally, one can find an herb farm online that sells fresh root in season, however.) Out of all these herbs, the only one I'd say you should definitely make fresh would be lemon balm. Dried lemon balm loses its potency fast, and as you'll learn a bit later, if you add one simple step to making lemon balm tincture, you'll have an excellent product.

The other ingredient you'll need is alcohol. It's best to get the highest proof that is legal in your state or province if you're within the U.S. or Canada. (If you're outside North America, finding a high proof probably won't be an issue; lucky you!) A good 190-proof grain alcohol such as Everclear or Golden Grain is best. If it's legal in your area, then definitely go for a brand such as one of these. The rest of us will have to make due with the highest proof grain alcohol or vodka available where we live. While the results are far superior with 190-proof grain alcohol, I have had good success with tinctures made from 151-proof Everclear, although the resulting colors of the tinctures are often more brown than the usual greens, reds, or yellows, etc., and the medicines are less potent than that coming from a good kick-in-the-pants alcohol.

And while we're discussing alcohols, let's get this right out on the table: If you're concerned about taking tinctures because of the alcohol content, fear not. The average tincture dosage has about as much alcohol as a ripe banana. Unless there is an alcohol sensitivity, alcoholism, or a religious conviction that means alcohol isn't even a consideration in your family, tincture is safe - when used properly. On the other hand, drinking the whole bottle is definitely inadvisable; but it usually tastes disgusting enough to warrant that won't happen.

When preparing a fresh herb tincture by using Simpler's method, chop the herb well and stuff into a clean, dry jar; but don't pack it in too tightly. Give the herbs a little elbow room. Fill the jar with alcohol until the alcohol is just above the level of herb. If the herb floats, you can use a weight such as a rock to hold the herb down, but only if you promise never to shake the jar. That's a quick and easy way to smash the glass.

Once you've combined herb and alcohol, store the jar in a cool, dark place and wait two weeks before straining out the herb. This being said, if you don't get around to straining for a week (or a year as I've sometimes done), it's no big deal. The alcohol preserves what's in there without fear of spoilage, and it does look rather stunning to see the plants floating in colored liquid. But two weeks is all that is needed, as nothing else will be extracted from the plant after that time.

If you're using dried herbs for your tinctures, you'll want to try and follow the ratios that are provided below. A two-week wait is again all that's required for a dried herb tincture to be complete.

After a lot of experimenting, I discovered that an old ricer I had in the back of a kitchen cupboard was the very best way to thoroughly strain all the tincture from the plant material. I've tried all kinds of fancy squeezy techniques in the past, only to discover the ricer offers the best leverage to a set of hands that can otherwise not open a pickle jar; even one that's been opened before.

When the herb has been strained, pour it back into the jar, cap it tightly, and label it with the date and the kind of herb. I also like to include information such as where the herb was purchased, grown, or wildharvested; what kind of alcohol was used; and what method I used, such as Simpler's or a particular ratio such as 1:5 (one part herb to five parts alcohol). You can also benefit from adding dosage information and/or your intended usage of the tincture.

Now let's take a look at the various tinctures you can make for your first aid kit. This list includes the Latin name of each herb, along with what part of each herb you should use for tincture making, whether dried or fresh. Dried herbs require a bit more manipulation, so ratios of herb to liquid are included. Occasionally, you'll notice the dried herb tincture requires a different dosage than the fresh herb tincture.

Boneset (*Eupatorium perfoliatum*)

Fresh Herb: Whole flowering plant. Dosage: 20 to 40 drops in hot water, up to three times daily.

Dried Herb: Tincture of dried herb not advisable.

Echinacea (*Echinacea purpurea*)

Fresh Herb: Root and flowers (or just root). Dosage: 30 to 100 drops, up to five times daily.

Dried Herb: Root and flowers (or just root), one part herb to five parts liquid (70% alcohol, 30% pure water). Dosage: One to two teaspoons, up to five times daily.

Feverfew (*Chrysanthemum parthenium*)

Fresh Herb: Whole flowering plant. Dosage: 30 to 60 drops, up to four times daily.

Dried Herb: Whole flowering plant, one part herb to five parts liquid (50% alcohol, 50% water). Dosage: 30 to 60 drops, up to four times daily.

Golden Seal (*Hydrastis canadensis*)

Fresh Herb: Root and leaves. Dosage: 15 to 30 drops, up to four times daily.

Dried Herb: Root and leaves, one part herb to five

parts liquid (70% alcohol, 30% pure water). Dosage: 30 to 75 drops, up to four times daily.

Hawthorn (*Crataegus spp.*)

Fresh Herb: Berries and/or flowering branches. Dosage: 10 to 30 drops, up to three times daily. Dried Herb: Berries, one part herb to five parts liquid (60% alcohol, 40% pure water). Dosage: 10 to 30 drops, up to three times daily.

Lemon Balm (*Melissa officinalis*)

Fresh Herb Only: Whole unchopped flowering herb, one part herb to two parts liquid (60% alcohol, 40% pure water) in blender. Blend until a slurry is produced, then jar and cap. Hint: Lemon balm is a sensitive plant that loses its oils easily. The less you handle it in its fresh state, the better. Best harvested on a dry spring morning. If you want to get extra particular, water the plant the night before and don't pick it if it's too hot the next morning. The more exact you choose to be with lemon balm, the better the end product.) Dosage: 20 to 40 drops as needed.

Passionflower (*Passiflora caerulea* or *incarnata*)

>Fresh Herb: Whole plant. Dosage: 20 to 40 drops, up to four times daily.
>
>Dried Herb: Whole plant, one part herb to five parts liquid (50% alcohol, 50% pure water). Dosage: 20 to 40 drops, up to four times daily.

Valerian (*Valeriana spp.*)

>Fresh Herb: Whole plant. Dosage: 30 to 90 drops, up to three times daily.
>
>Dried Herb: Root, one part herb to five parts liquid (70% alcohol, 30% pure water). Dosage: 30 to 90 drops, up to three times daily.
>
>**NOTE**: Both forms cause drowsiness. Do not use for more than a few weeks at a time, as it may cause depression with regular use, especially with the dried root tincture. Not for children.

Yarrow (*Achillea millefolium*)

>Fresh Herb: Whole flowering plant. Dosage: 10 to 40 drops, up to five times daily.
>
>Dried Herb: Whole flowering plant, one part herb to five parts liquid (70% alcohol, 30% pure water). Dosage: 10 to 40 drops, up to five times daily.

Preparing Your Kit

You've learned about various natural first aid remedies, you've prepared your own oils, salves, and tinctures, and now it's finally time to pull everything together so it's ready when you need it. What follows is a list of the standard non-herbal first aid gear everyone should have, along with some quick ideas for boxing everything up nicely.

Choosing Your First Aid Container

Once you have all your first aid gear together, you'll need something to keep everything in. It's best to organize things as compact as possible, but you also need easy access. It shouldn't resemble your kitchen junk drawer, for instance, or you'll never find the bandages when you need them. (You might, however, find a half dozen paper clips and a lost Christmas cookie cutter.)

You can always go out and buy something elaborate or extra sturdy, but repurposing an old container is an excellent idea. Even a shoe box will work to start with; just make sure it's strong enough and that things won't spill out all over the place if it's grabbed in an emergency. An old Tupperware container, an unused tackle box, even a file box or a crate with a lid will do.

Above all, make sure that whatever you choose is clearly marked and that everyone in your family knows what's in it and where you're keeping it (preferably out of the reach of young children).

Note: I know it's easy to go all out creative with it, but decorating your kit with lace, silk flowers, or pictures of your dog Tippy is not advisable. Even if Tippy is really cute and lowers your blood pressure in an emergency.

Standard First Aid Gear

There are a few basic items that every first aid kit should contain. Whether you decide to gather these up on your own or purchase a premade kit from the store is entirely up to you. There are some very reasonably priced kits in nearly any pharmacy (I've seen the most basic starting at only $5), and if you want the "big daddy" that even contains a set of defibrillator paddles, you can go straight to your country's official Red Cross website. But putting the items together on your own is an inexpensive way to go, especially if you have a discount pharmacy near you. Take along the following shopping list and grab your essentials.

- Bandages (assorted sizes)
- Absorbent compress bandages
- Roller bandages
- Gauze pads (3 x 3 and 4 x 4)
- Adhesive cloth tape
- Iodine
- Rubbing alcohol
- Instant cold compress
- Oral thermometer (non-mercury, non-glass)
- Tweezers

- Cotton balls and cotton swabs

Don't forget the following extras that you'll need in order to use your herbs:

- Tea ball or reusable muslin tea bags
- Eyedroppers for tinctures, if not included in your tincture bottles

Also remember to keep any official first aid instruction booklets in your kit, such as any Red Cross booklets and your print copy of "Nature to the Rescue".

Dried Herbs

The dried herbs we discussed for tea usage are as follows:

Angelica Seed (*Angelica archangelica*)

Boneset (*Eupatorium perfoliatum*)

Calendula (*Calendula officinalis*)

Cardamom Pods (*Elettaria cardamomum*)

Catmint (*Nepeta cataria*)

Chamomile (*Matricaria recutita*)

Chia Seed (*Salvia hispanica*)

Elder Flower (*Sambucus nigra*)

Elecampane (*Inula helenium*)

Feverfew (*Chrysanthemum parthenium*)

Ginger (*Zingiber officinalis*)

Hibiscus (*Hibiscus sabdariffa*)

Horehound (*Marrubium vulgare*)

Hyssop (*Hyssopus officinalis*)

Lemon Balm (*Melissa officinalis*)

Licorice Root (*Glycyrrhiza glabra*)

Marshmallow Root (*Althea officinalis*)

Peppermint (*Mentha piperita*)

Mullein Leaf (*Verbascum thapsus*)

Valerian (*Valeriana spp.*)

White Pine Bark (*Pinus spp.*)

Wild Cherry (*Prunus virginiana*)

Willow Bark (*Salix spp.*)

Yarrow (*Achillea millefolium*)

Remember, you don't need this entire list of dried herbs. Just make sure you have at least one good remedy from each chapter of the book. If you're trying to be economical, be sure to rely on the multipurpose herbs such as chamomile and peppermint.

I'm asked all the time about where to shop for herbs. If you don't have a reliable health food store in your area that stocks good, freshly dried herbs, there are several reliable online stores that supply them. A few popular choices with good reputations would be:

Frontier Co-op (www.frontiercoop.com)

Mountain Rose Herbs (www.MountainRoseHerbs.com)

Starwest Botanicals (www. Starwest-Botanicals.com)

Going with a small online store can be a great idea too; you can often find high quality homegrown herbs for good prices. Etsy is a nice way to find herb growers because you can check the ratings and responses of previous customers. But of course always use caution when shopping from a new source, and start out with a small order so you can check the product first.

I've also added several dried herbs, tinctures, and salves to my website store at www.DianeKidman.com/dianes-shop.html. It's not an all-inclusive list, but I do try and add some of the harder-to-find items people most commonly ask me about.

Once you've gathered all your dried herbs together, you'll want to package them for your kit. Anything that will keep about an ounce of each individual herb (or three ounces of tea blends) airtight and fresh will do. Small plastic resealable baggies, little glass jars with tight lids, even tins as long as they screw shut or are able to seal well. Mark the containers clearly with the name of the herb and the date it was packaged, and make sure to keep the herbs fresh. (Most dried herbs have a two- or three-year shelf life; I prefer to change mine over each year, just to be sure I have the best quality possible.) If there's enough room on the label without making it hard to read, you can also include steeping instructions and dosage.

Conclusion

Now that your herbal first aid kit is complete, I bet you're feeling pretty proud of yourself. You should be! You're ready for just about anything life can throw at you, what with all those herbs you've collected and remedies you've concocted. You're practically Florence Nightingale. If your kit looks especially wonderful, please do email me a photo at themommyspot@gmail.com. I'd love to post it at www.DianeKidman.com where it can inspire others to give herbal remedies a shot.

At this point, your best bet is to keep the kit topped up with fresh remedies and nearby at all times. Because I just saw your husband eying a pair of stilts in the back of your garage. And he looked pretty determined.

Bibliography

Briggs, Dr. Spike and Mackenzie, Dr. Campbell. *Outdoor Medical Emergency Handbook.* Firefly Books, Ltd., 2010.

Moore, Michael. *Herbal Materia Medica.* Southwest School of Botanical Medicine, 1995.

Moore, Michael. *Herbal Repertory in Clinical Practice.* Southwest School of Botanical Medicine, 1990.

Tierra, Michael, C.A., O.M.D., and Lust, John, N.D. *The Natural Remedy Bible.* Pocket Books, 2003.

Other books by Diane Kidman

Herbs Gone Wild! Ancient Remedies Turned Loose

Beauty Gone Wild! Herbal Remedies for Gorgeous Skin & Hair

Hair Gone Wild! Recipes & Remedies for Natural Tresses

Teas for Life: 101 Herbal Teas for Greater Health

Smoothie Power! Recipes for Weight Loss, Vitality, & the Occasional Superpower

All of these bestselling titles are available in both paperback and Kindle formats.

http://www.DianeKidman.com

htttp://www.dkMommySpot.com

Twitter: dkmommy

www.ingramcontent.com/pod-product-compliance
Lightning Source LLC
Chambersburg PA
CBHW070538290526
45790CB00002B/550

* 9 7 8 1 4 8 1 1 6 6 0 5 8 *